Ten
Commandments
for a Healthy Lifestyle

Ten Commandments for a Healthy Lifestyle

Use these simple principles and see miraculous
changes take place in your life!

Dr. Perry Wolk-Weiss

To order books or arrange speaking engagements, please contact:
The Get Well Center, PC
5 E. Union Ave. Bound Brook, NJ 08805
732-356-1155
www.getwellcenter.com

To order additional copies of this book, contact:
Xlibris Corporation
1-888-795-4274
www.Xlibris.com
Orders@Xlibris.com
46745

CONTENTS

Dedication

Any book is never the sole work of its author but is the collaboration of many dedicated souls. I would like to thank, first, my wife Cindy for her great insights and her ability to help me better define all of my creative ideas. In addition, I am grateful to my son Ben from whom I learn so much about going for my dreams; to my parents who taught me that I can accomplish anything; to my patients who have helped me understand how powerful the body is in healing itself; to Don and Silka for their support over the years; and to Jude Rittenhouse who spent long hours helping to edit this book.

ACKNOWLEDGEMENTS

I am grateful to the following for material used or referenced in this book:

American Chiropractic Association
American Heart Association
Anonymous author of the poem A Life's Journey
Richard Bandler & John Grinder: Neuro-Linguistic
    Programming
Dr. Cheryl Braselton Anderson
Anne Christiansen Bulers & *Consumer* magazine
CDC Resource Guide to Nutrition and Physical Activity & *The
    National Health and Nutrition Examination Survey*
Dr. Norman Cousins
Dave Dravecky for his book *When You Can't Come Back*
Albert Einstein-for being a smart person
Elizabeth Frazo
Google
Henry Gray's *Anatomy of the Human Body*
Allen Luks & Peggy Payne for their book *The Healing Power
    of Doing Good*
National Sleep Foundation
Hans Selye for his book *Stress of Life*
Lisa Sutherland, PhD., & Ira Dreyfuss, AP
Maria Fiatarone Singh, MD
Talmud
www.actsof kindness.com
www.focalpointyoga.com
www.nal.usda.gov (USDA web-site)
www.newstarget.com
www.Stretching.com

PREFACE

This inspiration for this book came about while I was engaged in the study of Integrated Kabbalistic Healing. This kind of spiritual work promotes introspection into what makes us whole beings and how we relate to reality. During one of the meditations, the concept of using the Ten Commandments as a framework around which to share much of the basic health information I have communicated to my patients over the years came about.

Using the Ten Commandments as a foundation is done with the highest respect for what is the true intention of the real Ten Commandments. We all have our own individual relationships with a higher power.

I have spent the last twenty-five years of my life helping children and adults to achieve wellness. By wellness I mean a balance between your body, mind and spirit. This book is an extension of that process. Hopefully the *Ten Commandments for a Healthy Lifestyle* will inspire you to examine those areas of your personal health that might be improved by implementing any one of the commandments I mentioned. If from reading this book you are motivated to make some changes in your life and it brings you greater joy then I have achieved my goal.

INTRODUCTION

When Moses climbed Mt. Sinai to receive the tablets with the Ten Commandments, what many people do not know is that there was an additional set of tablets given to him. God, being a loving individual, wanted to insure that humans had some guidelines that would help guarantee their health and well being, so God gave Moses the *Ten Commandments for a Healthy Lifestyle.*

These rules or guidelines are important if we want to enjoy a life of good health and well-being. There are no guarantees that, if you absolutely follow all of these rules, you will never have illness in your life. Many other factors, over which we have little control, also affect our health. Genetics, pollution, and stress are just some of these factors. So, to shift the odds in our favor, the more we follow the "Golden Rules" or *Ten Commandments for a Healthy Lifestyle,* the higher chance we have of enjoying a long healthy life.

Just imagine for a moment that you were invited to play a game of chess, yet no one ever explained the rules to you. It would be very difficult to win, let alone enjoy the game. The level of frustration for you and your partner would also be high, since you were never playing by the rules. During my years as a health care provider, I have tried to follow these rules as closely as possible. Unfortunately, being human, I am not perfect and sometimes stray. Usually my body will let me know, sooner or later, that I have strayed, and I will have to pay the price for "sinning." I also have enjoyed the benefits associated with adhering to the commandments. Over the years, I have had the privilege of meeting many different people and of being able to see the benefits for those who adhere closely to the rules; I have also seen the ill effects for those who stray.

You will ultimately have to decide for yourself how these commandments fit into your belief system. Since one of the many gifts we have been given is free will, you have a choice. So if you are tired of how your body feels and functions every day, then perhaps it is time to get back to the truths that Moses was given so many years ago. Hey, the guy lived a very long time. He must have known something we don't know!

COMMANDMENT I

Thou Shalt Breathe

For many years obstetricians would turn newborn babies upside down and smack them on the rear end to initiate breathing. That's kind of a strange and barbaric concept if you think about it. Thankfully, this is something that is not done today. Yet, the concept of how vital the breath is to our whole existence should not be minimized. Let's face it. If we don't breathe, we don't live.

What could be more essential than oxygen and the process that gets it into our bodies? But do we truly know how to breathe? Were you ever taught how to breathe in school? Of course not! We all take breathing for granted.

We generally take twelve to twenty breathes per minute. Breathing moves oxygen to all our cells. It helps in the flow of lymphatic fluid and allows for the discharge of poisons from our bodies. Modulating our breath can allow us to make beautiful music on a musical instrument.

According to www.focalpointyoga.com, a web-site on Breath Therapy, "in the average person, the breathing mechanism is functioning at only a fraction of its potential. When full free breathing is restored, every system in the body begins to work better. We find that the breath itself naturally heals and renews the body, mind and spirit. Conscious Breathing becomes a very powerful self-directed healing process. The breath reveals itself to be an untapped natural resource, a therapeutic tool, for health, growth and change."

The first step you can take to affect your breathing is to re-experience your breath for the very first time. As I said earlier, many of us pay little attention to our breath. Paying greater attention to our breath can place us more in the present moment because our breath is always in the present moment not in the past or future, where many of us tend to live, but in the present.

There are many different types of *controlled breathing* and ways to use our breath. In Yoga they talk about *Pranayama*. Loosely translated as prana, it means breath control. The ancient yogis developed many breathing techniques to maximize the benefits of prana. Pranayama is used in yoga as a separate practice to help clear and cleanse the body and mind. Re-learning how to breathe will add more energy to your system, increase calm emotions, release physical tension and help to increase health.

While sitting or standing with spine erect, inhale through your nose, filling the lower section of your lungs first as your belly expands. Then allow the breath to fill the middle part of your lungs, noticing how the ribs, breastbone and chest expand as you bring the life force into your body. Naturally allow this air to fill the upper chest and hold for several seconds. Exhale the breath slowly, and notice the belly contracting towards the spine. Try to do this in a smooth fashion and inhale for four counts, hold for two counts and slowly exhale for four counts. This begins to take on a rhythmic feel.

Another breathing exercise you may want to try is the alternate nostril breathing. This type of breathing balances the body and mind as it calms anxiety. You may also feel more alert after this practice. This is a good practice to use if you feel that late afternoon sleepy feeling around three or four o'clock:

1. Sit on a cushion or straight back chair with your head, neck and chest vertically aligned.
2. Using one hand, fold the middle, ring and pinkie fingers in towards the palm.
3. Gently close the left nostril off with the index finger and exhale fully through your right nostril.
4. Inhale through your right nostril.
5. Close the right nostril with your thumb and exhale through your left nostril.
6. Inhale through your left nostril.
7. Close your left nostril and exhale through your right nostril.

This is one full cycle. You may continue for twenty cycles, finishing this exercise by exhaling through your right nostril. You may also want to count the inhalation and exhalation so that they are even. Start with four seconds in and out, then you may build up gradually to about twelve counts per breath. Be mindful not to strain; this is to be done gently.

The best way to start is to keep things simple. Just begin by becoming aware of your breath and where it originates during different times of the day. Notice when you are stressed and the breath is high in the chest, or when you are relaxed and it is a full belly breath. Spend a few minutes of every day in solitude, focusing on your breath. Do this for fifteen to twenty minutes every day, and see if you begin to notice any changes in how your body functions and how you feel.

Homework:

Breathing Practice fifteen to twenty minutes each day. Several times during the day, notice your breath without judging yourself. Where is it in the body? Is it short and shallow, or relaxed and open? A great time to notice is before answering the phone, at a red light, standing in line at the market or the bank and before walking into your home after a day of work.

COMMANDMENT II
Thou Shalt Eat Nutritious Foods

Food—glorious, wonderful food! Eating and what we eat has become very big business in this country. Yet food, in its basic form, is really the fuel that runs this engine we call a body. The quality of the food we ingest determines the quantity of vitamins and other nutrients our bodies have available to use as fuel for repair and growth. Simply said: Poor Food, Poor Performance.

As a health care provider observing patients, I have become absolutely convinced that many of the health conditions that afflict Americans have a relationship to the quality and quantity of food we eat. According to an article titled: "High Costs Of Poor Eating Patterns In the United States," published by Elizabeth Frazão, an agricultural economist with the Food and Rural Economics Division of the Economic Research Service within the U.S. Department of Agriculture, I'm not the only one who has noticed this correlation. In her article, Ms. Frazão looks at the top causes of death in the United States—coronary heart disease, cancer and stroke—and their relationship to diet. She states that, "After accounting for co-morbidity and potential double-counting, it is estimated that healthier diets might prevent $71 billion per year in medical costs, lost productivity, and the value of premature deaths associated with these conditions."

It is not the occasional sinful dessert that causes these extreme health issues, but rather the consistently poor eating habits many Americans consider to be "a good diet." We each need to make conscious, careful, informed decisions about what we put in our bodies. When we do not, we can end up paying a shockingly high price.

We are all as different on the inside as we are on the outside. Trying to put everyone on the same type of diet makes no sense at all. Therefore, rather than give you the magic diet secret of the century in this commandment, I am going to share some guidelines that have held the test of time.

1. **Eat foods that are minimally processed**. Foods should be chock full of vital nutrients. Fresh fruits and vegetables should make up a large part of your diet, followed by whole grains such as brown rice, millet, quinoa and oatmeal; then legumes or beans such as soy beans, garbanzo beans, black beans, kidney beans, lentils and pinto beans. Dairy products such as eggs, milk and cheese should be eaten in moderate amounts and should be organic whenever possible. Finally, add meats such as chicken, fish, beef or pork, if you are so inclined. Being a vegetarian, I am biased. Frankly, I feel that most Americans would be healthier without meat-based sources of protein. Yet I also understand the reality of most people's eating habits; therefore, I recommend that if you consume meat-based proteins, do so in small amounts.

2. **Eat Organic as often as possible.** When I tell people this, I sometimes hear statements such as: "Is it really better? How come the organic products all look yucky compared to non-organic? It's so expensive!" I have heard this all too often. However, studies as early as 1993* showed that organic foods do have higher nutrient value than non-organic foods. Obviously, organic foods are also void of all the dangerous pesticides and chemicals that can do potential harm to our bodies. So I ask you to consider which is more expensive in the long run: organic food or high medical expenses?

    Organic food is more expensive, but so were radios, televisions, calculators, and computers when they first came out. Once the supply and demand increased, the prices came down. In the last three years, I have seen more stores offer organic products than ever before. The more you ask for organic items especially local organics, the more farms will produce and the less expensive these products will be. Besides, as my Dad often said to me, "You get what you pay for."

    Most supermarkets now offer organic produce. If yours offers none or does not offer enough, ASK! Supermarkets will meet customer needs if there are enough people requesting organic. So the more you request, the more you will get!

3. **Eat Less.** We can walk into any supermarket in the United States and be overwhelmed with the abundance of food choices. It does not mean we have to eat it all! Obesity is a huge epidemic in America, especially among children. Obesity can lead to such conditions as cardiovascular disease, hypertension, dyslipidemia (high fats/cholesterol), and type II diabetes. A good practice to get into is eating a larger meal either in the morning or afternoon and leaving dinner as the smaller meal. Most Americans are less active after dinner and, therefore, burn fewer of the calories they consume late in the day.

4. **Reduce the sugar content in your diet.** USDA advises people who eat a 2,000-calorie healthful diet to try to limit themselves to about ten teaspoons of added sugars per day. In fact, the average American does *not* eat a healthful diet, but consumes twenty teaspoons of added sugars per day. In 1999 Americans consumed an average of sixty-four pounds of sugar per person, per year. Mary Poppins may have said, "A spoonful of sugar helps the medicine go down," yet, with the amount of sugar Americans are consuming, they are going to be taking more and more medicine! Excess sugar in our diets certainly increases our chances of getting adult-onset diabetes, cancer, heart disease and becoming obese.

   Begin to read labels. You may be surprised to find out how much sugar is hidden in our foods. Any ingredient ending in "-ose" is a form of sugar. Take a look at what you drink and, if it is anything other than water, you will usually find high fructose corn syrup as one of the first ingredients.

   For example, this is the ingredient list for a popular ice tea drink: premium brewed tea using filtered water, high fructose corn syrup, citric acid, natural lemon flavor. It contains twenty-four grams of sugar.

   There are many other options for foods and beverages without sugar in them. For example, a simple soft drink alternative is to make your own sun tea by taking a bunch of herbal (fruity) tea bags, placing them in a clear jar of water, putting it out in the sun for a couple of hours, and you're done! Become more aware of your sugar intake, use your creativity and remember the old, true saying: "If you don't have your health, you don't have anything."

5. **Reduce your sodium intake.** The National Heart, Lung, and Blood Institute (NHLBI) continues to support the sodium and salt intake recommended by the National High Blood Pressure Education Program, which suggests that, as part of an overall healthy diet, Americans should consume no more than 2,400 mg of sodium a day. That equals about six grams of salt (sodium chloride).

Here is a checklist from the American Heart Association on how to lower your salt intake:

- Don't use salt during cooking. (Try a salt-free seasoning substitute.)
- Don't salt food before you taste it.
- Learn to use spices and herbs to enhance the taste of your food.
- Eat less salted potato and corn chips, lunch meats and hot dogs, salt pork, ham hocks, dill pickles and many canned foods. All of these have a lot of salt.
- Eat more fresh fruits and vegetables and less canned or frozen ones.
- Use fresh fruit and raw vegetables as snacks instead of chips or salted nuts.
- Look at food labels; many canned and frozen foods say "low salt" or "low sodium."
- Select unsalted nuts or seeds, dried beans, peas and lentils.
- Avoid adding salt and canned vegetables to homemade dishes.
- Select unsalted, fat-free broths, bouillons or soups.
- Select fat-free (skim) milk or low-fat milk, low-sodium, low-fat cheeses, as well as low-fat yogurt or soy/rice milk.
- When dining out, be specific about what you want and how you want it prepared. Request your meals be prepared without salt.

6. **Eat foods high in antioxidants.** What do small red beans, blueberries, pinto beans and artichokes have in common? They are all high in antioxidants. There are many other foods that fit this category; so, if you don't like these, there is no shortage of other choices. The USDA web site is a great source of information: www.nal.usda.gov. The USDA site lists nutrient content for many

foods as well as which foods are high in antioxidants. Antioxidants help to prevent free-radical development in your body. In simple terms, they keep your body from rusting out. Think of your body's "rusting" process as something similar to how sheet metal oxidizes and rusts, thus destroying a car. Now, remember that free radicals have been linked to cancer development.

7. **Finally, be adventurous.** Most people get into a routine and rarely change their diets. Try new foods and recipes. Expand your culinary horizons. If you can't cook, take a cooking lesson. Just as reading different types of books makes you well-rounded, eating different foods will light up your life. *Bon Appetit!*

Homework:

Pick any month and change your eating habits for that full month. Eat more vegetables and less meat. Eat smaller quantities that are made of higher quality ingredients. Reduce the number of carbohydrates you consume. Follow the guidelines I have outlined. Notice whether or not you see a marked change in your energy levels, waistline, or in how you feel overall. You can always go back to the same old diet you had before. Be adventurous. Who knows what might happen!

*   *This statement is substantiated by, among other things, a Soil Association study titled, "Food Quality and Human Health," published in 2001 in the United Kingdom's* Organic Farming*; and on an article titled, "Organic Foods vs. Supermarket Foods: element Levels," by Bob L. Smith, published in 1993 in the* Journal of Applied Nutrition, Vol. 45-1, *and copyrighted by the International Academy of Nutrition and Preventive Medicine.*

COMMANDMENT III

Thou Shalt Move

Before giving him the *Ten Commandments for a Healthy Lifestyle,* God said to Moses, "Get your people moving." Why do you think they walked for so long in the desert? It wasn't just to find the Promised Land; it was to develop a habit of exercise!

You have probably heard the saying, "use it or lose it." A sedentary lifestyle causes stagnation, weight gain and loss of vitality. The most recent estimates of overweight children in the United States are: ten percent of children age two to five years, fifteen percent of children age six to eleven years, and almost sixteen percent of children age twelve to nineteen years. According to the *CDC Resource Guide to Nutrition and Physical Activity,* these estimates were generated using weight and stature measurements collected in the 1999-2000 National Health and Nutrition Examination Survey (NHANES).

Lack of physical activity is a serious problem in the United States. As our world becomes more "modernized," we become less active. Consider this: the basic human body has not changed much over the last several hundred years. Evolution is a slow process. Yet the level of physical activity in which each of us is engaged has decreased considerably. In 1776, the year our country declared its independence, daily activities often consisted of physically plowing the acreage that fed your family, making most of your clothing by hand, building your own home and, while there were horses to ride, most people walked wherever they needed to go. They did not hop in their cars.

Many teens spend more time playing at their computers than they do at physical activities. Researcher Lisa Sutherland, PhD., of the University of North Carolina at Chapel Hill, analyzed federal data on the diet; weight and physical activity of teens age twelve to nineteen. Her research was summarized in the May 13, 2003 article,

"Inactivity Blamed for Teens' Weight Gains," by Ira Dreyfuss of the Associated Press. According to Dr. Sutherland's research from 1980 to 2000, the quantity of calories eaten rose one percent and obesity rose ten percent, while physical activity dropped thirteen percent.

If you're looking for the "fountain of youth" or the next magic anti-aging pill, exercise would be the ticket. In 1990, Maria Fiatarone Singh, MD, an Australian geriatrician, conducted the following study: she took ten frail, institutionalized volunteers age ninety (plus or minus one year) and put them through eight weeks of high-intensity resistance training. Over the eight-week program, they were able to show an increase in strength that averaged 174 percent. This remarkable difference occurred in a group of people as sedentary as you can get.

So get off that couch, put down the remote, shut down the computer or video game and GET MOVING! I know it's not always so easy. Believe me, I have days when I would rather stay in my nice comfy bed than get up at 6:30 AM to go exercise. So here are five tips I've found helpful in getting motivated.

1. Change your mind-set
"People tend to limit their activity level based on how they see themselves athletically," according to Dr. Cheryl Braselton Anderson, an assistant professor of pediatrics at Baylor College of Medicine in Houston. She says that, "To do vigorous exercise, like running, swimming, or cycling, or any type of physical activity, you have to see yourself as a person who does these things."

A technique you can use to help change how you view yourself is called reframing. This technique works to alter the meaning or value of something by altering its context or description. Reframing is a powerful change stratagem. It changes our perceptions, and this may then affect our actions. This technique is part of Neuro-Linguistic Programming (NLP), which was developed by Richard Bandler and John Grinder in the 1980's.

How do you use reframing to get you motivated to exercise? You shift your focus and find a new way to envision exercise in your mind. Let me give you an example. Suppose you often look at exercise as something tedious and hard. When you think about exercise, all you see is yourself going through torture while you do it. As human beings, we're naturally motivated toward pleasure rather than displeasure. So, now, begin seeing not the work *during* the exercise but rather the end result. Start seeing into the future. How will you look in three or six months? Visualize your body looking slim, svelte and buffed. Think about all the energy you will have. Begin planning what your life will be like when you are fit. As you do this and continue it regularly, a reframe will take place in how you look at, or perceive, exercise. Then those early mornings (or whatever time you decide to exercise) won't seem so hard.

2. Chunk It Down

This idea comes from a time when I was in Dallas, Texas, for a seminar. I often like to exercise early in the morning, before the learning starts. Spending eight hours sitting in a seminar might exercise my brain, but my body gets itchy for movement. On this particular morning I chose to go for a run. Coming down the elevator, I met another chiropractor attending the seminar. As we talked, we decided to go running together, so we could continue our conversation.

During our run, I found out he was training for a marathon. I had occasionally thought about running a marathon; however, as fast as the idea came into my head it went out again. The notion of running a marathon, including all it would take to train for it, seemed overwhelming to me. While I do enjoy running approximately two to three miles, I don't think I really would like to run twenty-six miles. Yet, what my colleague said to me that day is something I want to pass on to you. He said the idea of running a marathon was overwhelming to him, too. What he did was "CHUNK-IT-DOWN." He never looked at the overall mileage he had to run, but rather broke it down into smaller amounts upon which he could build. Then the idea of running a marathon was within his capabilities.

You might not run a marathon, but you can learn to break your exercise goals into smaller components and then expand as you progress. This is rather like the saying: "How do you walk a thousand miles? One step at a time!"

3. Move The Blood & Air

Whatever exercise activities you chose, you need to make sure to get your cardiovascular and respiratory systems working. You need to have an aerobic component to your exercise regime that lasts a minimum of thirty minutes. Running, brisk walking, bike riding, tennis, cross-country skiing and swimming are just a few of the exercises that get the blood and air moving.

4. Become Gumby

As we age the biggest change, besides wrinkles, is a loss of flexibility. That loss often contributes to an increase in injuries. To avoid this, you need to be involved in a regular (and I do mean regular) stretching program. It does not take long before a pause in one's stretching program leads to muscles and ligaments tightening up. Yoga is great for increasing flexibility. A good book available on stretching is titled, *Stretching*. The book was first published in 1975 and can be found at the web site, www.stretching.com or in local bookstores. It is well illustrated and can give you great ideas on how to stay flexible. I also discuss this topic further in commandment ten.

It only takes fifteen minutes per day of stretching to maintain flexibility. If you eliminate one situation comedy that you watch on television, you'll have more than enough time to stretch or stretch while watching that comedy!

5. Have Fun

There is nothing that is going to kill any exercise habit faster than not having fun while you are doing it. Find an activity or combination of activities that you enjoy and that meet the criteria above. For example, I really enjoy tennis. Varghese has been my tennis partner for several years, and we take turns at winning. Even on the days when I am not playing my best, I still enjoy the game and look forward to going back the next time to do better. MAKE YOUR EXERCISE FUN!

Homework:

Designate fifteen minutes out of your daily routine to take a walk. Then build your exercise habit from there.

COMMANDMENT IV
Thou Shalt Hydrate Thyself

Our bodies are estimated to consist of about sixty to seventy percent water. Blood is mostly water, and our muscles, lungs and brain all contain a lot of water. The brain is composed of seventy percent water, and the lungs are nearly ninety percent water. We need to drink water because water is required to regulate body temperature and to provide the means for nutrients to travel to all of our organs. Water also transports oxygen to our cells, removes waste and protects our joints and organs.

Juice is not water, coffee is not water and soda is not water. Only water is water! While the other drinks contain water, the body has to process it to remove the H_2O molecules that exist in the drink. Nothing hydrates you faster than plain water.

When speaking with patients about hydrating themselves, I am often asked about sport drinks (such as Gatorade™). While sport drinks do have the ability to restore electrolytes and supply the necessary carbohydrates to working muscles, they should not be used to replace water in the average person. Unless you are an athlete involved in serious athletic competition or training, you should not make these your regular liquids for hydration. Your body needs a liquid with no agenda—nothing attached to it—and water fits that bill. If you'd like to read more about this, go to: http://www.NewsTarget.com/001959.html ("Gatorade, soft drinks, coffee and alcohol no substitute for body's health requirement for pure water, says doctor").

Should you drink tap water, bottled water, flavored water, or smart water (this water they must send to college)? Which is the best for you?

According to "Bottled Water: Better Than the Tap," an article by Anne Christiansen Bullers, published in the July-August 2002

U.S.F.D.A. *Consumer* magazine, Americans drank a whopping five billion gallons of bottled water in 2001. This article indicates that bottled water is highly regulated by the F.D.A. and, therefore, must meet certain criteria concerning the levels of contaminants. Very often these levels are the same levels established for tap water. It appears the overall consensus is that tap and bottled water are very similar in their level of safety. The only place there appears to be a difference is in the taste. The manufacturers of flavored water and smart water might make a lot of claims; but I, personally, do not see the value. So the decision is truly up to you and your pocketbook. What is most important is getting the water inside you.

Now, how much water should you drink? This is not an easy question to answer, since we all have different needs based upon age, body type, and level of physical activity. By doing a search of various health-related papers and web pages, I found that the consensus of opinion points to about one-half ounce of water per pound of body weight for minimally active people; this translates to about eight to ten eight-ounce glasses per day. Athletes should consume closer to thirteen or fourteen eight-ounce glasses per day. One must also take into account the level of humidity, temperature and how much one sweats. The bottom line is to regularly hydrate your body and don't wait until you are thirsty to drink water.

Homework:

Drink Up!

COMMANDMENT V
Thou Shalt Rest

ZZZZZZZZZZ. Oh excuse me! I was just resting. With the hectic lives many people lead in America, recent articles have shown that many of us are sleep deprived. According to a National Sleep Foundation 2005 Annual Sleep Survey:

- About seven in ten adults are getting less than eight hours of sleep a night on weekdays.
- Sleep problems are more prevalent among those who report getting "a good night's sleep" only a few nights a week or less.
- Those who report getting less sleep than they say they need to function at their best are more likely than those who get more sleep than they need to have missed work or events or made errors at work at least one day in the past three months.
- A large majority (75%) report having had at least one symptom of a sleep problem a few nights a week or more within the past year.
- One-half of all respondents (50%) report feeling tired, fatigued or not up to par during wake time at least one day a week, with 17% saying this happens every day or almost every day.
- Those with sleep problems are twice as likely to feel stressed and tired.

Sleep is vital for the body to renew and revitalize itself. This is recharging time—a chance for the body to be focused on healing and cleansing, without the distractions that occur during our waking hours. The human body has only so much energy. Think of it like your cell phone battery. If you have your cell phone on and do not talk, it uses less power and the battery can last longer. The more you speak on your cell, the faster the battery discharges. Either way, there is only a limited amount of energy the battery can store and release. The battery, like your body, needs to be hooked back up to its re-charger. For your body, sleep is that re-charger.

Besides, if you do not sleep you will miss out on all the wonderful dreams that humans experience. Just imagine all the places you can go and people you can meet in your dreams, whether or not you can remember them (and, if you don't remember them, it may be because you are sleep deprived).

So how do you make sure you get the proper rest you need?

1. **Make an intention**. Just as you might set a goal to eat less or exercise more, you need to make an intention to get enough sleep. Create a set time to get to bed. You do not have to feel compelled to stay up late watching the hundreds of channels now available on cable or satellite television! Besides, how many infomercials for the latest gadget can you watch?

2. **Exercise.** Regular exercise can help to dissipate much of the stress that builds in your body during the day. This stress can often make sleeping at night difficult, since your mind and body try to wrestle with all that stress. Exercise helps you release energy and relax.

3. **Slow Down**. For many people, life is so hectic during the day either with their jobs, commuting or taking care of a family they literally just collapse right before bed. Make it a ritual, during those fifteen minutes before bedtime, to meditate, take a warm bath, sit quietly or just read. Do something to allow your body and mind to transition to sleep. Sometimes even focusing on your breath can be helpful.

4. **Have the correct equipment.** What equipment do you need to sleep? A comfortable bed is the most important thing, obviously. What type of bed and how do you pick the correct mattress? Should you get a firm, extra firm, extra extra firm, super duper deluxe hard-as-rock firm, or one of those new air-adjustable ones, or maybe the new space-age super-foam mattresses? It truly can get confusing. Here are some general guidelines that I often share with my patients.

   • *Decide on what you can afford.* Mattress costs can vary from around the $750 range to above $5,000. While a bed is something in which you spend a significant amount of time, you'll want to be realistic. Once you decide on how much you are reasonably going to spend, then you can make better choices when you go shopping for a mattress. The Internet is a great place to window shop, but you still have to try out beds.

- *Take the bed for a test drive.* You would never buy a car without testing it out first. You should not buy a bed without first trying it out. If you sleep with a partner, make sure that person comes with you. What is good for the gander is not necessarily good for the goose, as the saying goes. Everyone has different needs, and you both have to come to a mutual decision based upon sleeping habits, height and weight. Take the time to lie on mattresses in the store for several minutes. Some stores may allow you to take them home for a thirty-day trial.

- *Not all beds are created equal.* Firm for one manufacturer may not be the same in another manufacturer's line of beds. So ignore the firm, extra firm designations and, as I said previously, try them out. What you do want is a SUPPORTIVE mattress. One that conforms to your natural body curves and MAKES *YOU* FEEL COMFORTABLE!

- *Do not be fooled by names.* "Orthopedic," "Chiropractor approved" and "medically approved" are just hype for more sales. You are better off inquiring about the guts of the mattress than to be sold on the associated names they put on mattresses. Most of the major manufacturers are good options to consider because they typically stand behind their products.

5. **Sleeping Positions**. To properly support your spine, you should preferably sleep with a single pillow beneath your head and supporting your neck. The primary job of the pillow is to support your neck, not your head. I personally use a water pillow made by Chiroflow™ and also sell them to my patients. I get great feedback about the pillows, although there are many other fine pillows on the market. Using one pillow, rather than multiple pillows is important because it places your head in the correct position for maintaining the natural curve of the neck. If you sleep with more than one pillow, you may risk reducing the natural curve of the neck, which can lead to future problems. If you have a breathing

problem, try elevating the mattress or getting a gradual foam bolster, so the angle on your neck is still maintained.

You should sleep either on your side or your back. Sleeping on your stomach causes you to twist your head in order to breathe and this causes torque of the neck muscles. Sleep is the only time the neck muscles get a chance to rest after carrying around those bowling ball heads of ours. Yes, our heads weigh approximately eleven pounds—the weight of a small bowling ball. Use of pillows under your knees is fine when you have a lower back problem. If you're pregnant you have my permission to sleep in whatever position you find comfortable!

One final note about rest: make sure you do what you need in order to feel refreshed each morning. Life is too precious to sleepwalk through it. Nor do you want to be so tired that you put your health or the people you care about at risk by doing something such as driving while fatigued. So go take a quick nap.

Homework:

Stop watching TV thirty minutes prior to bed and spend the time sitting quietly meditating, focusing on your breath. You can also do this lying in bed.

COMMANDMENT VI
Thou Shalt Serve

Dr. Norman Cousins has said, "If something comes to life in others because of you, then you have made an approach to immortality." The *Talmud*, a vast collection of Jewish laws and customs, says, "All men are responsible for one another." To be of service feeds our souls. When we give of ourselves unselfishly to help others, it often comes back tenfold.

I have been fortunate to see the Dali Lama of Tibet on two occasions. The first was in New York's Central Park and the second was when he came to Rutgers Stadium in New Brunswick, New Jersey. Each time, the primary thing I noticed was his sense of peace as he shared himself with the hundreds of people attending his lecture.

Being of service to others is something that can change our internal physiology. In an article appearing on the Acts of Random Kindness Foundation's web site (www.actsofkindness.org), there is a reference to Allen Luks' and Peggy Payne's book, *The Healing Power of Doing Good*. Luks is the former executive director of the Institute for the Advancement of Health and executive director of Big Brothers/Big Sisters of New York City. Luks and Payne researched thousands of "do-gooders" to discover what they might experience from being of service to others. What the co-authors found was that many of the volunteers experienced a "helper's high," a physical and emotional sensation of euphoria that lasted for days or weeks and spread into other areas of the volunteers' lives. More importantly, they found that the good feeling returned when people even mentally recalled their experiences of volunteering. Furthermore, these researchers also found that the more people volunteered, the more benefits they received.

In fact, more than ninety percent of Luks' and Payne's volunteers reported that regular volunteering produced euphoric feelings.

Such feelings are a powerful antidote to stress, which creates negative effects on our physiology. Long-term stress can raise blood pressure; contribute to heart disease, diabetes and many other health maladies. Hans Selye, the Hungarian physician who wrote the 1956 groundbreaking book *Stress of Life*, emphasized that any activity, which gives us a sense of positive accomplishment, becomes stress reducing.

It is not unusual for older adults who have lost a spouse to experience a sense of depression and loneliness. Finding even just one day a week to give unselfishly—to focus on helping another person—can significantly impact a person's sense of purpose in this world.

During my career as a chiropractor, many of my mentors have commented that, in order to be successful, we cannot be solely focused on the financial gain from the work we perform. To be truly successful, we must be focused on being of service to others, and then the financial rewards will come.

Are you being of service to others? What areas of interest do you have that you could use to help others? Are you a reader? Perhaps you could help teach people to read or read to those who have vision impairments. Are you good with fixing things, doing carpentry? Perhaps you could volunteer for Habitat for Humanity. Passionate volunteers are in short supply. I am sure there is some organization out there that you could connect with to serve others.

Perhaps your way of being of service is to commit to doing random acts of kindness. Simply make a decision to be more kind and compassionate to people you meet every day, whether you know them or not. Try it for a couple of months and notice how you feel. I bet it will release a few endorphins in your body, so eventually you will be hooked. Not such a bad habit to have!

Homework:

Spend one week or even one day looking for ways to perform random acts of kindness. Certainly do this for other people in your community, but do not forget yourself. Pay attention to your thoughts and devote one day to having only kind thoughts towards yourself. Work on removing self-judgement when negative thoughts arise.

Commandment VII

Thou Shalt See Life As A Journey

You will leave this world the same way you came: with nothing. Enjoy all that happens in your life, yet hold onto nothing.

Wise words, yet letting go is never easy. Life is a very complicated endeavor. We often get caught up in our daily activities—taking care of a family or working at a career or job—and we forget that life truly is a journey we only get to experience once.

Several years ago, when my wife and I were on vacation, we decided to take a canoe trip down a local river. Rivers rarely ever go in a straight line, and this one certainly was no exception. As my wife and I meandered down the river, we never knew what scene would await us as we came around a bend. Each time we glided around a new turn in the river, there was a surprise. Life is much the same: we never know what is around the bend, so we might as well enjoy the journey.

I know that, for many people, life seems very hard; and for other people it seems like everything goes their way. Sometimes the difference boils down to choices. When hurricane Katrina devastated New Orleans, it turned people's lives upside down. This is an example of how we have little control over some of the events in our lives. Yet we do have control over how we chose to respond to such events. We have free will: the ability to decide how we will perceive and respond to what happens in our lives. It has been said that we can make a heaven of hell or a hell of heaven; the choice is up to us.

Here's a poem I came across that inspired me and may also speak to you:

Life's Journey

Do not undermine your worth by comparing yourself with others.
It is because we are different that each of us is special.
Do not set your goals by what other people deem important.
Only you know what is best for you.
Do not take for granted the things closest to your heart.
Cling to them as you would your life; for without them, life is meaningless.
Do not let your life slip through your fingers by living in the past nor for the future.
By living your life one day at a time, you live all of the days of your life.
Do not give up when you still have something to give.
Nothing is really over until the moment you stop trying.
It is a fragile thread that binds us to each other.
Do not be afraid to encounter risks.
It is by taking chances that we learn how to be brave.
Do not shut love out of your life by saying it is impossible to find.
The quickest way to receive love is to give love.
The fastest way to lose love is to hold it too tightly.
In addition, the best way to keep love is to give it wings.
Do not dismiss your dreams.
To be without dreams is to be without hope.
To be without hope is to be without purpose.
Do not run through life so fast that you forget not only where you have been,
but also where you are going.
Life is not a race, but a journey to be savored each step of the way.
~Anonymous

When giving my workshop on stress management to corporations, I often quote from an article written about Dave Dravecky. Dave was a major league baseball pitcher who lost his arm to cancer. He became depressed not only from the ordeal associated with the surgery but also from the shattering of his boyhood dream: to play in the major leagues. He was depressed enough to even consider suicide as an option. But what Dave finally realized was that God had a bigger mission for him. In his book, *When You Can't Come Back*, he shares how he realized that, while it is good to plan for the future, you can't live there, because there is too much treasure in a day. What we can learn from Dave and others like him is that each day is a gift, a treasure, something to be cherished. We need to truly practice being in the moment.

Have you ever had a time when your child was young and asked you to play? Maybe it was throwing a football, having a tea party or riding a bike; and during the entire time you were with this child you were thinking about the six million things you had on your to-do list. Ask yourself: was I truly present with my child? Once any moment has passed, we can never get it back. We all need to stop living in the future and the past. They are gone or have not yet arrived. Begin, now, to live in the present and realize: this *is* the journey.

As we progress through our lives, we are creating memories. With time passing by so quickly, our memories will be something that sustains us as we age. What kind of memories are you presently living? Your experience of today—this moment in time—will be your memory of tomorrow. A friend of mine once asked, "What will be your dash?" The dash is that space between the date you were born and the date you pass from this world: 1955-20??. What will happen in that dash for you? How will you perceive it? Take a few minutes out of your day and decide what kind of memories you are living. The homework exercises below will help, and they'll also help you become more present.

Homework:

1. Begin each day with a sitting meditation. In the beginning you may only be able to do five or ten minutes. For many people, the concept of sitting and doing nothing in silence is hard. Just like anything else, it takes practice. When you sit, try and bring your awareness to your breath. Become gently focused on it as if it is the only thing that exists for you right now. When a thought comes into your mind (and it will) just imagine you are dropping it into a small brook, like a leaf falling from a tree, and watch it being carried away. Then come back to your breath. This will help you get used to being in the present moment.

2. When you are performing tasks during the day, become aware of how present you are with what you are doing. Do you eat a meal while reading the paper or a book and realize you have no concept of what you just ate? Try to spend one week fully experiencing your food when you eat meals. Be totally present during the eating process. Enjoy the tastes, smells and textures of the food. My wife, who teaches Mindfulness Based Meditation,

uses an exercise with new students to help them become more mindful. She gives them one raisin to eat and has them fully, slowly experience the eating of that raisin.

3. Listen to the church bells and birds. Near my office are several churches and one of them plays bell tones periodically during the day. When I hear this, I like to think it is a signal to stop and pay attention. You can use many things in this way: the ringing of the phone, the call of a bird, even a stoplight or stop sign as you drive. Simple, yet these can be little reminders during our day to tune into where we are and ask ourselves if we are fully present. Take a moment and touch your breath and come home to yourself!

COMMANDMENT VIII
Thou Shalt Nurture Thy Spirit

We live at a frenetic pace. Allowing time for meditation and reflection fosters a quiet, peaceful mind. Break this rule and psychological health suffers. When psychological health suffers, the body ultimately suffers, too. This is one aspect of what is meant when you hear about spirit, mind and body being one interconnected whole.

Take a moment and consider what the phrase nurturing your spirit means to you. If you pick up many of the magazines that target women, you will often see articles discussing how to nurture your spirit or inner soul. So, before you can nurture your spirit, it seems logical that you would want to have a grasp on what that means for you.

To me it means listening to my little inner voice—the voice that tells me when I am tired, when I am stressed, when I feel overwhelmed. It's important to listen and pay attention to this voice rather than ignore it, because these subtle messages help me get in touch with who I am at the core. It's not easy. It takes work and guts—guts to truly separate my true self from what people expect of me, what they think I should be, what they thought I would be or what they needed me to be in order to save or rescue them.

This book is an example of nurturing my inner spirit. For a long time, I had this desire to write a book. I am not a writer by profession (something you may have figured out by reading this far) and did not want to write the great American novel. I just thought it would be fun to write about something I know—something that could benefit other people.

It could be easy for me to say, "Me write a book? Who am I? Deepak Chopra, Dr. Mehmet Oz, or some other great guru?" I could procrastinate and do the "someday I'll . . ." routine. Well, someday rarely ever comes. I am not even sure, as I am writing, how this will turn out. Yet, I decided that I had to at least start, and even if it does not become a great work and only gets read by my immediate fan club, I will at least have been able to satisfy a personal desire. I will have honored the inner spirit in me that brings me joy when I listen to it.

How do you nurture your inner spirit on a daily basis? Do you make time for what is truly important to you? Do you have a desire to paint, write, learn a musical instrument, be an actor or perhaps travel? Find what truly, deeply in your heart gives you joy and find a way to make it part of your life. I am not suggesting that you selfishly pursue something at the expense of others you love. However, if you don't honor your inner spirit, you and those around you will be impacted in a negative fashion.

Do you remember the show "All In The Family," where Carol O'Connor played Archie Bunker and Jean Stapleton played his wife, Edith? Archie would frequently say to Edith, "Stifle it!" when she was about to speak her mind. While she held the family together, Archie rarely let her truly express her inner spirit. Is that the kind of life you want?

In the previous commandment, I mentioned using some meditation techniques to help you become more present. The homework for this commandment will help you explore how meditation can help you nurture your spirit.

Homework:

Commit to a minimum of fifteen minutes during the day—or at least once per week—when you can spend time totally alone. Try to find a place that is quiet—a place where you feel peaceful. You might go for a walk in the woods, or just find a place in your home that you can call your "sacred place." Make this a place where you will not be disturbed—no phones or any other distractions.

You can close your eyes or keep them open, whichever feels right to you. Preferably sit rather than lie down, since many people will fall asleep when they are lying down. You do not want to disassociate from this process by falling asleep.

Begin to focus on your breathing. Just become aware of your breath. You can have some quiet music on in the background if you'd like. As you increase your awareness of your breath, also increase awareness of your body. Breathe out any tension you might feel.

In the beginning your mind will be a noisy place. It probably will never totally quiet down. Just allow the thoughts to wash through, like a leaf falling into a stream and being carried away. If you get into the habit of this process, you will allow your inner voice to make its presence known. By creating this sacred time and space, you are signaling that you are ready to listen.

Sometimes it helps to just start with a question such as, "What brings me true joy in my life?" Sit quietly and trust that the answer will come.

You are opening space in your life to tap into the infinite consciousness, also known as heart consciousness. This process will help you hear your inner spirit. Remember, your answers may not come in words. Be open to whatever comes and be ready to receive surprises.

Some people find that using this quiet time to journal their thoughts helps them get in touch with their inner spirit. Do whatever feels right and works best for you. Just, please, do not go through your life without honoring who you truly are. God created someone special, a one-of-a-kind human being: YOU!

COMMANDMENT IX

Thou Shalt Nurture Thy Nervous System

We experience EVERYTHING through our nervous systems. Nothing happens in our body without the brain telling it to happen.

Many people have probably given little consideration to the importance of keeping the nervous system healthy. I am sure you have considered exercise, diet, your cholesterol number and perhaps even mental fitness. Most people take better and more consistent care of their teeth than they do of their spine and nervous system. Yet, neglect your nervous system, a vital part of your body, and everything can fall apart. As far as I am concerned, this is the keystone to good health. Let me explain.

Take a moment to consider your body and how it truly works. The brain is the central computer that literally coordinates the functioning of all tissues, organs and systems in the body. According to Henry Gray, who wrote the classic 1918 text, *Anatomy of The Human Body*, "The **NERVOUS SYSTEM** is the most complicated and highly organized of the various systems which make up the human body. It is the mechanism concerned with the correlation and integration of various bodily processes and the reactions and adjustments of the organism to its environment. In addition the cerebral cortex is concerned with conscious life."

In the human embryo, the brain and nervous system are among the earliest organs and systems to develop. When you grow from two cells to approximately 100 trillion cells and ten major organ systems, there is a lot of coordination that has to take place—and that's just the first project the brain and nervous system complete! Right now, you're reading this text while your heart beats at seventy-two beats per minute. Your lungs are exchanging carbon dioxide and oxygen, while you are digesting your food (if you have recently eaten), and you are reading at the same time. Meanwhile, your postural muscles hold you upright and your immune system fights miniature battles. WOW! That sure is a lot of stuff to do without giving any of it a single conscious thought. All of this is brought to you by your amazing and wonderful central nervous system.

Your brain is the major coordinator/computer with the spinal column extending off of it like a large cable, and then smaller nerves branch off to smaller ones, etc. Just think, you can poke a pin into any area of your skin and feel it. This happens because of the extensive network of sensory nerves.

The spinal column protects and allows the delicate nerves of the spinal cord to exit and carry messages. However, the vertebrae of the spine can misalign or subluxate with all the physical, chemical and emotional stresses we encounter. Often subluxations go unnoticed in the early stages. When symptoms do show up, many people do not associate the symptoms with a vertebral subluxation. When we do not take care of our spines with regular chiropractic care, subluxations of the spine cause nerve interruption and eventually lead to lack of harmony, also known as Dis-Ease.

Vertebral subluxations might also be called nerve interference. Here's an example. One of the most common complaints patients present in my office is a headache. It can be anything from a tension-type headache to a full, head-exploding migraine. One day my assistant had one of those horrendous migraines that makes you want to literally die. As I began to work on her, one of the misalignments I discovered was a specific type of subluxation related to the sacrum. The sacrum is the triangular bone at the base of your spine where your tailbone attaches. Once I realized the sacrum needed correction, a simple painless adjustment restored the normal motion, and her headache pain began to subside. Most physicians would never associate something like this with migraines. The most common scenario would probably have been to heavily medicate the patient and possibly run a slew of tests, which would not have shown what was causing the headache.

Vertebral subluxations disrupt the normal communication system in our body and block the flow of innate intelligence that gives us life. All of us, from infants to adults, need our spines checked by a good chiropractor. Not everyone needs an adjustment to his or her spine. This is just like good oral hygiene; that is, everyone should have their teeth checked, but not everyone needs to have them drilled, filled, pulled, realigned with braces, etc.

Keeping your spine free of subluxations and having a nervous system that flows properly can do more to help you stay healthy than most people imagine. I have personally witnessed (and received) the benefits of good, regular chiropractic care. The migraine story above is just one very small example of hundreds of patients during my twenty-five years in practice that have changed their lives because of chiropractic. There are many conditions that respond well to chiropractic care other than the typical aching back or sore neck. Asthma, allergies, digestive complaints, dizziness and fatigue are just a few additional examples of conditions that can develop from spinal misalignments.

One more thing: if God did not want you to see a chiropractor, God would not have made them!

Homework:

If you have not done so, schedule an annual visit to your chiropractor. If you don't have a chiropractor (and aren't able to come to New Jersey to see me), ask friends, co-workers or neighbors. A referral is the best source. Other resources would be the American Chiropractic Association, or look on the web for your local state chiropractic association.

COMMANDMENT X
Thou Shalt Remain Flexible

A regular program of stretching our bodies is essential. Lack of stretching stiffens the joints and ligaments, increasing the chance of injury. Also, remaining flexible in our thoughts and our ability to accept new ideas prevents us from becoming stiff in our mindset.

If you observe the cattails or reeds by an open salt marsh, you will notice how flexible they are when the strong winds blow. It is this built-in flexibility that helps the reeds survive in their environment without breaking. So, too, must we be flexible in body, mind and spirit to prevent us from breaking when the strong winds blow through our lives and environments. I'll begin by discussing the flexibility of the body. Then, I will end this last commandment by discussing the flexibility of the mind and spirit.

If I were to ask you to describe someone seventy-plus years of age, you probably would not use the word flexible. You might even say that such a person seemed stiff compared to the mobility of someone half his or her age. When patients come to me in pain, they often say they feel like a ninety year old. While we do tend to loose flexibility as we age, as a result of changes in collagen—the elastic fibers that make up our ligaments—we do not have to become "stiff as boards." Maintaining our flexibility is essential to preventing injuries. It can also be a major asset that determines how we experience our lives.

Flexibility in our joints, muscles and ligaments is a result of creating a consistent habit of stretching. If you have lost flexibility, you can gain it back. One of my tennis coaches described how, early in his tennis career, he was so inflexible that when he was sitting on the floor with his knees bent he could barely pull them apart. After getting involved in a regular program of yoga and stretching, he was able to easily move his knees to the floor. He shared this with me while I was watching him perform some pre-practice stretches. He was fifty-nine years old and more flexible than most of the other players at the practice who were younger.

I personally can attest to the power of consistent stretching to help improve flexibility. While I am no contortionist, I have experienced the benefits of stretching, particularly with yoga. Having a consistent yoga practice has certainly increased my flexibility. When I do not do yoga, I feel stiff and lethargic. One particular series of yoga poses I like is called the Sun Salutation. I attempt to do Sun Salutations at least three days a week. It is great because the postures are so versatile. They can be done quickly or slowly, held for long periods of time or short, and can vary depending on your level of flexibility. Before I play tennis or go for a run, I try and do a set of Sun Salutations.

The Sun Salutation contains twelve postures that flow one into another. There is also a breathing pattern associated with this exercise since the breath, or Prana, is vital to our life function. If you do a Google™ search for Sun Salutation, you will find many different web-sites offering examples, including directions and pictures.

There are differing opinions about the best times to stretch. Some say to stretch after the muscles have warmed up. Others say to stretch after vigorous exercise. The Sun Salute is gentle enough to allow you to start off slowly and then progress as your muscles warm up. I prefer to begin with gentle stretches and then increase the intensity as I get more blood into the muscles. If you were performing intense physical activity, like training for a marathon, I would recommend you stretch afterwards as well, in order to prevent the muscles from tightening. Just begin to make stretching a consistent habit and you will truly love the results. Be patient and it will happen.

In conclusion, I would like to discuss the flexibility of the mind and spirit. In the early days, or the "good olde days" as some would say, the world was smaller and simpler. With advances in transportation and the creation of the Internet, the world has become much larger, and access to information has increased exponentially. In the field of health care and healing, we still have not even scratched the surface in understanding the healing potential of the human body. The mind-body-spirit connection is just beginning to evolve as a study of how our body truly works. Quantum physics is allowing us to have a greater understanding about the connection we have to everyone and everything in this universe. Consider this concept: the molecules of air you breathe today are probably the same molecules of air that your neighbor has inhaled and exhaled. Since energy and matter are never destroyed, they just change form. Your body contains the matter from other creatures that have roamed the earth.

To think that drugs and surgery are the only path to health and vitality is a very nearsighted view of the human potential to be healthy. If we are truly going to enjoy a life that is full and vital, we must begin to develop a flexible mind. We can consciously notice and then set aside our initial habit of being skeptical about things we do not understand. I do not mean we need to naively believe everything we read or see. Instead, I suggest that, when we come across a notion that is outside our typical paradigm, we can ask, "Could this be possible?" Then we can investigate and see how the notion stands up to the laws of nature. What if the Wright brothers had said, "It's impossible for humans to fly like a bird?" Where would many of us be if it weren't for Dr. Martin Cooper? Who is he? He is a former general manager for the systems division at Motorola and is considered the inventor of the first modern portable handset, or cell phone, as we now know it.

In the next century, change in many areas of our lives is going to happen so rapidly that the majority of us will not even be able to keep up with it. Having an open and flexible mind, particularly where your health is concerned, can make the difference between living a life of sickness and disease or a life of vitality and wholeness.

In my chiropractic practice, I see miracles occur every day, particularly when I'm caring for children. Despite the fact that their parents—and certainly the young child receiving the treatment—have little understanding of how the healing takes place in their bodies, it happens.

Homework:

Begin cultivating an expansive mind. Read books and magazines. Attend lectures about subjects that you might have some interest in but do not fully understand. Discuss new concepts with friends and family. Open to the possibility that you may not know everything and neither do the doctors. Consider this quote by Albert Einstein:

"The most beautiful thing we can experience is the mysterious. It is the source of all true art and all science. He to whom this emotion is a stranger, who can no longer pause to wonder and stand rapt in awe, is as good as dead: his eyes are closed."

Flex your mind and your body. You'll be amazed at the places they will take you!

STAYING THE COURSE

If you are reading this part of the book, hopefully you have read all the commandments and have not just skipped to the end! One of the biggest obstacles to achieving change in our lives is staying the course, or keeping our focus. It is the person who never gives up, no matter what obstacles are thrown in the way, that is the person who achieves his/her goals.

Tony Robbins, author and motivational speaker, often talks about why people maintain behaviors that do not assist them in obtaining what they want out of life. He feels that we have become hardwired toward activities that provide us pleasure, and that even the bad habits we continue to perform over and over again are giving us pleasure in some way. Since human beings naturally try to avoid pain and seek pleasure, we develop neural associations in our brains around certain activities. These neural associations can go back to early childhood. For example, over-eating is certainly something that, if continuously done, will eventually harm our health. Yet many people, despite the pain over-eating might cause them in the future or even in the present, continue because somewhere they have linked in their mind more pleasure from over indulging than from eating in a healthy way. This neural pattern (that is, the association we have made with food) needs to be shifted in order to change the habit.

Taking the time to read *The Ten Commandments for a Healthy Lifestyle* is the first step in the process of changing old habits. But all of the information will be useful only if we also begin to raise our awareness of what might be limiting our abilities to put into practice the ideas and strategies shared in this book. When we step back and look at our lives, we can often find additional areas where we had valuable information to make our lives better, yet we never implemented these plans—we let them fall by the wayside after our initial start.

How do we have the self-awareness and courage to step back and see the truth, when the truth is that our old ingrained habits are not really giving us pleasure, rather they are causing us pain?

This can be subtle and difficult to see when the pain is not having the energy to enjoy our families, or not achieving the life dreams we had, or incurring healthcare expenses taking care of a dis-eased body. Sometimes our pain is simply a higher level of frustration than we deserve—something that can be almost invisible to us. So how do we make the change? How do we change habits, so that our behaviors serve us and help us live up to the commandments in this book?

First, make a decision: decide with passion from the heart that you no longer want to continue down this path. I remember watching Popeye cartoons as a kid and, just when Popeye was getting fed up with Blutto for tormenting him, just before Popeye ate his spinach, he would say, "That's all I can stand and I can't stand no more!" That is usually when all hell broke loose and Popeye saved the day. It's time to decide that you can't stand it any more!

Next, take a look at reality. What is creating the resistance that prevents you from exercising regularly, or eating properly, or honoring your spirit, or any of the other commandments of health? What have you associated with these behaviors? You might want to grab a piece of paper and just journal your thoughts and feelings about why you over-eat or don't exercise (or whichever behavior seems to be an obstacle for you). Write down, without having any initial judgments, all the feelings and thoughts that come up for you. When you are finished writing, sit back and look at what you have written about each behavior. Often, simply becoming more aware of what lurks just under the surface of our daily lives and thoughts can help us to shift behaviors. Try to go a step further and use your new awareness to discover other patterns you could implement to replace old habits that no longer serve you.

For example, let's say you never find time to nurture yourself. Somehow, you are always doing something for everyone else except you! The kids, your spouse, your job—they all seem to come first; and, maybe, if you have time, you will do something for you. Perhaps you have always had a desire to paint, and never seem to find the time. There's always something getting in the way. The truth is, there is always enough time to do the things that are important in our lives. The truth is that we too often abdicate our own desires in an attempt to care for those we love (and, sometimes, even for work associations or even strangers). Our adult behaviors emerge from deep in our psyches.

So taking care of others can be a result of times when, as children, we were put in situations where one or both of our parents were either unavailable or ineffective, so we had to take care of our siblings' needs or even a parent's needs. Even marvelous parents can't always be there for us in all the ways children need.

Many people find it difficult to do this type of deep self-exploration alone. After all, relationship is a fundamental human need. So, for some people, it might be more useful to try working with a psychologist or Art Therapist or Integrated Kabbalistic Healer (or other professional) rather than trying to manage a deep inner exploration on their own. However you proceed, once you can see reality clearly, you can interrupt old patterns and make some different choices in your life.

Start small, pick one or two of the commandments and decide, on a scale of one to ten, how they are working in your life. If you feel you're close to a ten on one commandment, then move on to the next. If a commandment is appreciably less than a ten, then this is an area of your life to explore and revamp. Look at why this area is not working for you. Using the ideas I mentioned earlier, explore and then begin to create a plan of change. Search for ways to start associating pleasure with this commandment, then keeping on track with it will become easier. Make a game out of it. If you enjoy challenges, you might even try making a bet with your partner or a friend. We all like to do things that are fun, so create ways to make it FUN!

Track your progress and, when you feel you are well on your way towards making this commandment a stable part of your life, move on to the next. Give yourself time; strong oaks don't grow strong over night. Be compassionate with yourself. You may slip, get off track and divert from your path. Sometimes things happen that we do not expect. However, once you have associated pleasure with a commandment, you will get back to it very soon. Remember old habits are hard to change. Start TODAY!

PRODUCT SOURCES

Chiropractic and Holistic Health
American Chiropractic Association-*www.amerchiro.org*
Nambudripad's Allergy Elimination Technique-*www.naet.com*
International Chiropractic Pediatric Association-www.icpa4kids.org
American Holistic Health Association-www.ahha.org

Aromatherapy mists
Sarah's Essence Aromatherapy-http://www.sarahsessence.com

Meditation Resources
Center for Healing Journeys-www.centerforhealingjourneys.com
Center for Mindfulness at the University of Massachusetts Medical
Center www.umassmed.edu/cfm/index.aspx

Spiritual Support
A Society Of Souls-www.kabbalah.org

Food and Dietary Information
The World's Healthiest Foods, a book by George Mateljan, website: www.
Whfoods.org